The Greatest Discovery
in History
of All Mankind

by

Gerd Maximovič

(With strong help by **Shelby Vick**)

Table of contents

The Coué method is simple.
But all great things are simple.
This method is simplest,
So it is the greatest.

1. Introduction

In all religions there is the command of prayer. Who do you pray to? To God. Religion means: "religere", that is: connecting you with God. You will find this everywhere. In Christendom, in Islam, in Eastern religions, everywhere. Now, are they fools, worldwide and through all times registered, who insist on your praying each day five times, like in Islam? Or who declare: the most important thing for you to do each day is your praying (consuming only the shortest time) as the German reformer Martin Luther told us?

Fools, spreading this deep felt certainty throughout time and all over humanity? You can read it for instance in the Bible, Jesus Christ working miracles. You find written proof: the happening of "miracles", not only in Lourdes or Fatima, but in all times, and everywhere, and namely today as well. In religion (connecting us with God) they say this is due to Christ, Allah, Buddha, Manitou. Well, this may be. But you know, God is everywhere and He deems servant of all, of you and of me. His grace is not confined to any religion. He, God, is never hostage of any clan. God is graceful everywhere.

Imploring God through prayers works, they all know. Being Moslem, Christ or whatever you may be - prayer works. So, obviously, there must be a God-mode in us to fulfill many of our dreams. In former times they said, this is our Soul, connecting us with God. Nowadays, in modern times, we say, it is our subconscious to do this job. No matter which term you use, no matter, which religion you prefer, no matter who you are or where you live: true is, this kind of prayer works.

So, now let us have a look at the conditions and the circumstances of this which seems so incredible, but is so true, fundamentally.

First, some proof.

2. Shelby Vick

Looking around, you find everywhere witness of the infallible method of Emile Coué. First, let us have proof that it works. This proof is delivered by persons, being seriously ill, getting by spiritual means well again.
Look at this quotation:
"This is the faith that Jesus meant when he said - 'Thy faith hath made thee whole.' This is the faith that is responsible for the miracles of Lourdes, for miraculous healings everywhere. It matters not whether you be Catholic or Protestant, Jew or Gentile. Desire and faith such as these will heal you.
A month or two ago I read in the newspapers of a farmer, blind for two years, who went out in the field and prayed, 'that he should receive his sight.' At the end of the second day, his sight was completely restored. He was a Protestant. He went to no shrine - just out under the sky and prayed to God."
(Robert Collier: The Secret of the Ages. 1926. p. 149)

So, first, what is of interest, is the proof. I asked Shelby Vick, well-known author and editor of eMagazines, to give me at least a few lines on his own results in this respect. Before this we had a voluminous exchange of eMails on this and other themes.
He, Shelby Vick, kindly sent me this:
"Being a long-time believer in the power of positive thinking, I paid a lot of attention to Coue's book on auto-suggestion when it first came out. Over the years, it dwindled down to recalling 'Every day in every way, I'm getting better and better.'
Then, through Planetary Stories ⁻ ww.planetarystories.com - I had a renewal, thanks to Gerd Maximovic who is an avid follower of Coué.
Well, I had a major medical setback in the middle of 2015. Lost a lot of weight, blood pressure became quite erratic and, most important to me, extreme lethargy settled over me like a smothering blanket.
Gerd encouraged me to use auto-suggestion, and I started. In a couple of weeks, the lethargy lifted! Also, I began to gain weight.
Then I had another problem arise. Glaucoma has destroyed the vision in my right eye, and weakened my left one. Well, that became so bad that I could only read email with the aid of a magnifying glass, and forget reading normal books and magazines.
I adjusted the saying to: 'Every day in every way my eyesight is getting better and better.' No emphasis on any word, just plain repetition.

It worked!

Oh, it wasn't overnite. After a couple of weeks, I could detect a minor improvement. That was enough encouragement for me to keep going. In fact, it is not unusual for the process to take two weeks of repetition before results are noticeable.

Well, I can now read email and even read books! There is still trouble with tiny print or hazy electronic entries, but the improvement is a very good step in the right direction, so I will definitely continue! (My eye doctor was amazed at my improvement, but I let him think he deserved the credit for it

– even tho he had not begun any new treatment.)

Thinking back over everything, it came to me this is similar to programming a computer. The difference is it' s the subconscious which Coué' s discovery programs.

Looking back in history, this is not at all like the Shaver Mystery hooplah or Dianetics - - it's something you can easily prove for yourself.

Following you will find overwhelming examples of the success of Couè's process, and explanatory details. The goal is to establish belief in your mind to validate this revolutionary - yet simple! - procedure. You can read on or, ir you're already willing to accept the operation as a verified tool for self-improvement, you can start now. For instance, where I said 'eyesight', you can substitute your problem, repeat it twenty times at least four times each day. In two weeks, you will see evidence of success." (Shelby Vick)

3. Rules and Sayings

Can we help ourselves, being sick? Yes, we can, and we can do more than is usually conveyed. This is the method Emile Coué (among others) developped, and it is most important. Emile Coué was a French pharmacist. When he gave out medics to his patients and customers he realized: he could just hand over the medic without saying a word. Or he handed it over adding confirming words: "that's good", "that works", "it is healthy", and so on. Result: when he spoke positive words the situation of the patient was much better than when he remained silent. But why? What made the difference?
Obviously it was his words, his speaking, his positive confirmation. So, there is another factor, he concluded, regarding our health. This factor, shortly taken, is our subconscious, which can be impressed. And which heals us in all cases, working over night or over time. But Coué learned, we can influence our subconscious, in both ways: the good one or the bad one. Thinking positively (I am healthy and sound) or thinking negatively (I am sick and ill). Both ways work. Both ways!

Everything you really believe will become reality, within the limits of possibilities! Thinking positively (for instance: "I am well and sound"), you will be well and sound. Thinking negatively (for instance: "I am ill, I have acquired all diseases possible"), you will be ill.

What does this mean? It means, our personal subconsciousness is NEUTRAL, it realizes what you really think or know. Thinking positively, your way goes up, thinking negatively, your way goes down.
So, you can influence yourself (your own subconscious), no matter how old (or young) you are. It always works! But, dear reader, please mind, if you are a beginner it always takes time until your personal subconscious has learned that there is a new, positive "I" above, giving new positive rules.

This is, in short, what Emile Coué tells. Of course, everybody must read Coué himself. He is encouraging and his rules are strict and clear (the affirmations must be positive and short). Most important is his book "Autosuggestion". There are only three of his excellent books. Read them all!

Why am I so sure that Coué is one of the ablest und greatest men who ever lived? In 2005 I read one of his books ("Autosuggestion") and tried it out - and look: it worked! It was fascinating! Incredible! Then I watched German television for more than one year, each broadcast on sickness, healthcare and so on. Result: In more than a year, Emile Coué and his Autosuggestion never was mentioned. Not one time. Never. His books in German translation sell hundreds of thousands, but on German television he does not exist.

Afterwards I read more on this fascinating subject and learned: all of this thinking is based on German idealistic philosophy (Hegel, Schelling, Fichte and others); but these German philosophers did not realize that their ideas could be of practical value. The first one to give hints on the method of healing oneself through positive thinking was Immanuel Kant. The first one being really important to make these ideas practical was an US-American (who else, I might add, the country of the practical, efficient men who usually ask "What can I do with it?"): his name Phineas Parkhurst Quimby (1802 - 1866). He had a lot of pupils who learned from him. But there are others, men (and women), who made the same discovery, their own way, for instance as Emile Coué.

In short, this is a method additional to normal therapeutics (they are valid), but this additional method can work "miracles"! Yes, miracles! I learned in this respect that more than 100 (one hundred) US-boys und US-girls who suffered severely were cured this way as Coué describes. They regard it as a "miracle" to recover from severe disease. In result they (more than one hundred) founded all a church of their own!

In this respect, Emile Coué's texts are best, they are concise, encouraging, and his rules are simple and clear.

In all literature regarding "Autosuggestion", they say, this maybe may be the greatest discovery in history of all mankind. And, dear reader, I tell you: it is the greatest discovery in history of all mankind!

This method resembles the Mantrams used by Buddhists. Please, believe me, it works! You must know it or believe it! Because your subconscious realizes everything you really think. Our personal subconscious is a part of God. So you see, God is everywhere. God is in us. And God is Good, when you think positively!

Now follow the ideas conveyed by Emile Coué to us. Exactly, that means, well, 90 % of the following comes from Emile Coué, 10 % I picked out of other literature. But so we see, of course, Emile Coué is of highest importance!

How do you influence your personal subconscious? How did Emile Coué do it, and how did he learn about the great power of his method, being hidden within us? As mentioned above, he told his customers in his pharmacy: "This medicine is good, it is healthy!" And it worked. So we use the same method. We are telling ourselves (telling our subconscious) positive sayings on our health and welfare.

What shall a saying Emile Coué recommends look like?

Important (all due to Emile Coué): do not name your illness, else a wrong impression could enter. Express yourself definitely in a way as if your wish has already been fulfilled. And it will be realized, if possible under human conditions ever possible. This way "miracles" can happen. Remember the 100 New Churches mentioned.

These sayings must be short and positive. Very important therein is REPETITION. Repeat your sayings, repeat them, repeat them, repeat them. Use them in a childlike, monotone, automatically, without any stress. Read them from a slip of paper you have typed in and printed out on the computer.

Make this a routine, in normally reading this slip of paper. You read (whisper) it: mechanically, childishly, without any exertion (says Emile Coué). So the wishes sink best into your subconscious. Your effort is minimal, and the result is maximal.

Reading the sayings is possible, whispering them is better. Because your personal subconscious all day is busy with a lot of problems. When you whisper, the ideas you are proposing, they sink in better. But silently (and quickly) reading the slip of paper or recalling the sayings just from memory is also possible, and will work well. This depends on where and when you use the sayings. Standing in a subway train among a lot of people, better do not whisper, silently thinking the sayings there will do it.

What sayings should be on the slip of paper (or being stored in your memory)? Most important is the fundamental saying by Emile Coué, which you must always use and include in your individual list of sayings, it is this:

"Day by day, in all respects, I get better and better."

Or: "Day by day, in every way, I get better and better."

That's all. And you will get better and better!

Now, other sayings depend on your individual problems, of course. For instance, when your memory is not best, use this saying: "My memory and concentration are getting better and better!"

You sometimes feeling cramps in your legs or in your arms? Use this saying: "My arms and legs are always good, sound and relaxed."

And they will become what you wish, and will be!

Whatever is ailing you: put a short and positive saying against it, and your personal subconscious, your best friend and helper, will take care of it.

Please mind, 70 % of all diseases (severe diseases included) can be fought this way. Obviously there remain 30 % of all diseases for which you need the help of the normal doctor and the normal medicine. So, if it is not urgent, first try your sayings, and you oftentimes will witness a wonder: what seemed to be or to become a disease is gone.

And, of course, most important, using the standard saying by Emile Coué ("Day by day, in all respects, I get better and better") you can prevent most of all diseases without your knowing of them. But your subconscious, your best friend and helper, knows and will prevent them.

Make this a routine. This routine should not be bothering, it must be no burden, but shall be a slight addition to your normal activities. Although it is an easy, simple task, the result is enormous. That means, your on the slip of paper noted ideas (wishes) will sink down to your subconscious, and will be realized, if within the domain of the reasonable ever possible. You will gain a lot through this small acting which seems ridiculous, but is not. It is the greatest discovery in history of all mankind!

Martin Luther, the German reformer, said: never stop praying. And Emile Coué tells us: Never stop your sayings, for all of your life! That is correct! So we see how important just words (or ideas) can be.
You are feeling unwell, you do not know which disease it could be? You say doctors do not know the reason? That is of no importance. Use Coués standard saying ("Day by day, in every way, I get better and better"). Your subconscious finds out by itself which disease it is and will cure it without

your knowledge (says Emile Coué, one of the greatest men who ever lived).

 How to handle your slip of paper containing the sayings you want to see realized? Pull out the slip at certain times and read it three (or 10 or 30) times (depending on urgency). For instance after rising, after dinner, after supper, before going to bed. Most important: use it before your napping and sleeping, because when you sleep your subconscious has all time of the world, and works best. Make this a fixed routine, and you will see the results are like heaven sent!

Let us repeat it: using the Coué sayings is like prayer. Herewith you tell your subconscious what you want to be realized. Prayer, as mentioned above: Due to the Koran you shall pray five times a day. Luther, the German reformer, again, said: never stop praying; the most important thing you are doing all day over, is praying (that is establishing your connection with God). So do this "praying". In modern times it is just reading or whispering this slip of paper containing your sayings. This routine (reading the slip of paper) should be arranged in a way that it takes only a minimum of time.

Important, once more: don't name your illness, else a wrong impression could enter. I state again, express yourself definitely in a way as if your wish has already been fulfilled. And it will be realized, if under human conditions ever possible. This way "miracles" will happen.

Sleeping. Let us repeat this as well. When people are sick or unwell each doctor tells them, best thing you can do is sleeping. But why? Simple reason: because we all have a personal subconscious. It works best in sleep when it is not so much demanded as on day. Because in daytime there are much more problems to be watched and solved by our personal subconscious. At night time (we are sleeping) it is abundant free to work on our health.

There are two ways Emile Coué (among others) suggests: a) sayings or b) pictures, imaginations.

a) sayings, like above described.

b) pictures, imaginations: for instance a person, having cancer, imagines cancer as a lump in a picture, and then the person in its imagination "sees" how the lump is shrinking and shrinking, till it is totally gone.

Dear reader, choose your own way. Sayings (a) is the easier way, I guess.

Imagine, you often have spare time. For instance, standing in the kitchen, waiting for your repast getting ready, there are left over two or three minutes. Or you want to see the news on television, so you are waiting for two minutes. In this spare time you better read silently your slip of paper, that's far better than looking out of the window. So, printing out a slip for the kitchen, and one for your easy chair in front of the television set should be reasonable and effective.

Success is sure in 70 % of all cases of illness (severe diseases included). Now, please mind, being successful, there is a minor problem possible, due to Coué. You started your sayings, highly delighted you register success. But then there could be a little setback in the condition of your healing. Because the old ill conditions existed for many years in your mind and therefore are deeply rooted in your subconscious. A little setback need not happen, but maybe is possible. So, should it occur, there is no reason to panic (says Emile Coué). Then just use the same method (sayings), and you will recover utmost quickly. This time (the second time) your proceedings are far better and quicker, because you are used to it. The utmost possible, says Emile Coué, is a second setback. Then you can leave behind an illness which you finally will have defeated. Why am I mentioning a setback? When we are prepared for such a possible setback we can act much better. Then we are prepared, we are stronger. But, of course, there need not be a setback.

Am I too optimistic? No, I know from experience what I am reading and writing about now for ten years, in this respect. There are other reports in this text (Vick, Macnaghten, Kirk) you should very well consider.

Independence. Let us note again: we have a personal subconscious. We can influence it positively or negatively. It depends on us. Very important: this personal subconscious is partially INDEPENDENT, as they say in esoteric literature. And that is true! It is partially INDEPENDENT! It works ON ITS OWN. It gives us inspirations and ideas and reminds us of a lot of things because it never forgets anything. So, in short, it is a part of God within us. Being a part of God, it is neutral and depends on our positive or negative thinking.

Our personal subconscious is our BEST FRIEND AND HELPER, they say in esoteric literature. That also is true! That means, God is on our side! But please mind, God is on our side only when we think positively.

Question: Why does it work in each religion as well as outside of creed?

Answer: Responsible is our personal subconscious, it accepts everything we believe. Everybody, no matter what religion, has a personal subconscious. It realizes health for everyone, no matter what his creed. Call Allah, call Mary, call Buddha, it's not important whom you call - so the easiest and best way is to implore on your BEST FRIEND AND HELPER, your subconscious, of course.

What about God? The English and German languages are very interesting concerning God. In English there is a parallel: God = good, in German as well: Gott = gut. This is correct when you think positively. This is wrong when you think negatively, as stated above. So in result, God is good AND evil! Both! It depends on you, how YOU, dear reader, approach "Him", it depends on your thinking. As already stated, God in reality is NEUTRAL, and it is up to us if we approach "Him" positively or negatively. Our thinking proves it: we can tumble into illness, or we can rise out of it. Just through words or thinking.

A part of God within us? Yes! An ACTIVE part, please, mind you! Then, in consequence, God is the big subconscious. And great God as well is neutral. That means, God is good or evil, it depends on us, what we make out of "Him". Again, it is so important: It is good to know through experience that God (or Goddess or It or Whatever you want to call It) is on our side. But, please, do not forget, Goddess and God are neutral, so it is up to us to decide which aspect of a neutral Goddess or God is on our side! It's OUR choice. It's OUR thinking!

4. Hugh Macnaghten

Hugh Macnaghten: "Emile Coué, the man and his work" (1922). The author visited Coué in Nancy and took part in his lectures.
Here some quotations out of his book:

"M. Coué ... is never tired of affirming that he works no miracles, all he claims is that he is able in most cases to help us to cure ourselves. 'I cannot help you', he would say, 'if you have broken an arm or a leg; in that case you will go, if you are sensible, to a surgeon; but I may be able to help you to recover the use of a limb or an eye which from the mere fact of long disuse has ceased to act as a limb or an eye in being.'" (p. 4)

"... what you think, in the sphere of possibilities of course, tends irresistibly to become true for you." (p. 5)

"... indeed, we may sleep if we will, for our subconscious mind never sleeps and never forgets, and so his words sink in." (p. 6)

"... without effort. As soon as we nestle on the pillow we are to close our eyes and recite without stress, but just audibly, the well-known formula some twenty times: 'Every day in every respect I grow better and better' ... It seems childish, does it not? It is really childlike, and that is a very different thing." (p. 7)

"There was also present another girl who, for twenty years, had been blind in one eye. The blindness was the result of a blow when she was only three years old; for a time the eye was really blind; when it recovered, its little mistress had learnt to do without it and therefore never thought of using it, though it was ready to be used. After twenty years, some six weeks before our visit to Nancy, she had come to M. Coué and had been taught to see. The eye which, through no fault of its own, had been idle for twenty years has not yet quite caught up its more active mate, but it was not far behind and has possibly made up the lost ground by now." (p. 10 f)

"Sometimes ... specimens of elderly humanity present themselves, but M. Coué seemed hardly less hopeful of age than of youth, and no one was sent empty away. It is never too late to hope for amelioration even if complete cure is impossible. Old age is not a fatal disability: M. Coué makes no secret of his own sixty-five years, but hopes to work harder in the next ten years than even he has ever worked before." (p. 12)

"... that not the will but the imagination is the supreme force: always, however, the first step lies with the will, which before it abdicates must set

16

the imagination working in the right direction." (p. 18)

"... M. Coués teaching. Self-mastery based on recognition of the power of the imagination is the thing that matters. Quite unsensational is the truth which M. Coué brought home to most of us, and it is this: there is no need of miracle, but much need of the simple common sense which is so sadly uncommon." (p. 18 f)

Macnaghten quotes Horace:

"And none but he who watches them from birth,

The Genius, guardian of each child of earth,

Born when we're born, and dying when we die,

Now storm, now sunshine, knows the reason why."

And writes thereupon:

"The second quotation is the standard passage (i.e., our main source of information) on that elusive and mysterious person whom the Romans called the Genius. What exactly do we learn from this passage about this Genius? First, he is always with us from birth and dies with us; secondly, he rules our life; thirdly, he is so important as to be called (in the original) the God of human nature; fourthly, he dies when we die; fifthly, he is liable to change his expression; lastly, sometimes he looks bright (literally white) and sometimes black. If all this is true, our Genius must surely be a very remarkable person and we ought to know something about him. What fun it would be if the Genius, of whom Horace was writing some years before Christ was born, should prove to be an alias of the very modern sub-conscious self." (p. 27 f)

"Clearly we do not consciously direct the various processes on which our life depends: we do not look after our digestion or our breathing. If we take thought for either of these we shall make a sad mess of it, but, if wo do not take thought for these things, who does? Very certainly someone is busy looking after them, and on the whole he does his work well, expecially when we are young. If he does his work badly we suffer at once because then everything inside us begins to go wrong; hence come gout, constipation, insomnia, in short the whole miserable crowd of sicknesses." (p. 28)

"Always then remember that there are some ills which you can cure for yourself without expense far better than anyone else can cure them for you at vast expense..." (p. 29)

"Now, luckily, this unconscious self is most anxious to please you; he is also very impressionable, and at every moment is influenced by you, so that if you say or even think, 'I am ill', unfortunately for you, he always believes you, and then things all go wrong, just as, when you said or rather thought, 'I am quite well', everything, thanks to him, went on quite well inside you." (p. 29 f)

"Every morning before rising and every evening as soon as you are in bed, you must shut your eyes, so as to concentrate your attention, and repeat twenty times consecutively, moving your lips (that is indispensable) and counting mechanically on a string with twenty knots in it, the following phrase, "Every day in every respect I am getting better and better.'" (p. 32)

"But the rest of us will find M. Coué's is the easiest and safest way, especially as absence of effort is indispensable." (p. 33)

"M. Coué ... he has trusted himself when others laughed at him; he has waited for recognition till he was over sixty; he hasn't lied; he hasn't hated; he hasn't looked too good or talked too wise." (p. 36)

"Some people regard M. Coué as the founder of a new religion. It is a mistake. M. Coué is the apostle of common sense... he would say to us, 'Be Protestants or Catholics, be Bhuddists or Mohammedans, be what you will: it does not concern me whether you are zealots or Freethinkers: I only desire that all of you, from every point of view, Catholic, Nonconformist, or Agnostic, may grow daily better and better.'" (p. 38)

"... and M. Coué says expressly 'there is no miracle at all.' It is true that when a paralytic is cured on the spot, when he rushes to the window of the little upper room in Nancy, when he shouts to the people who are gathering for the next conférence in the courtyard below, 'Je marche, je marche', our thoughts go back nearly two thousand years to the beautiful gate of the Temple where a certain man, lame from his mother's womb, at Peter's word, leaping up, 'stood and walked and entered with them into the Temple, walking and leaping and praising God.' But the resemblance between the New Testament miracles and the work of M. Coué is superficial, the distinction fundamental. I do not know, though I think I know, what M. Coué would say about the passage I have just quoted: of the paralytic cured at Nancy every one knows that he has said it was no miracle; indeed for M. Coué ... miracles do not exist. The cures which are so astonishing as to seem miraculous are everyday occurrences." (p. 39)

"Blind men were cured, just as a girl blind of one eye was cured at Nancy..." (p. 43)

18

"But as a matter of fact the will does not abdicate until the imagination has in obedience to the will been startet in the right direction. If the imagination can do the rest, what sense is there in the will interfering any more? Point the rifle and pull the trigger of course, but surely it will be unwise to try and guide the bullet with your hand!" (p. 48)

5. Questions and Answers

Many authors bring correct items on Emile Coué's methods, and, unfortunately, mix them with wrong ideas. So, here, in short, a few things maybe to arise as questions, and the answers, partially already given above.

Question: "Is this Coué-method general valid, so that I can heal every thinkable disease with it?"
Answer: "No, up to 70 % of all diseases can be healed with it. Severe diseases included. That is a lot. So, being or feeling sick, first try the Coué-method, if it is not urgent."
Question: "What to do with the other about 30 % of diseases?"
Answer: "Regarding the remaining 30 %, visit the normal doctor. But even when you suffer of one of these 30 % please remind, the healing process always is performed by your subconscious. So, in any case, use your sayings, and your regeneration will run quicker and better."
Question: "What about drugs and medics?"
Answer: "Take them, when the normal doctor prescribes them."
Question: "Can I dismiss the normal doctor?"
Answer: "No. Never dismiss him. Remember the 30 % of diseases. And, please mind, the normal doctor is necessary, so the normal pharma industry is necessary as well."
Question: "Several authors say, using Coué's method I need no more bodily exercise. Is this correct?"
Answer: "This is not correct. Use your bodily exercise as usual. For instance biking, jogging, climbing, swimming, what ever deems right."
Question: "Having problems with my body, say with my teeth. Will it suffice to use the Coué method, and all these problems will disappear?"
Answer: "No, you always must consider two aspects. Your subconscious can have strong effects on your body, but this hinders not to use the usual means. So brush normally your teeth, and at the same time use the proposed sayings. This is valid for all other things regarding cleanness, sanity and so on. Use your soap, take your showers and at the same time - through sayings or through prayers - use the invisible forces exercised by your subconscious. Never forget the great invisible power within you."
Question: "What about my mind? When I use the positive saying regarding my memory and concentration, is there any additional mind activity necessary?"
Answer: "You must treat your mind exactly like your body. So use usual mind exercises. For instance read books, learn languages, write stories, publish magazines."
Question: "Someone told me the Coué method does not work. He tried it out, and it did not work with him. Is this person right?
Answer: Yes, this person can be right.
Question: But, another person told me, he tried the Coué method out, and it works very well with him. Is this person right?
Answer: Yes, this second person is right.
Question: But how comes, one person says, the Coué method does not work,

and it really does not work with him. And another person says, it works very well, and it really works well with him. How is this possible? Both persons offer contradictory opinions, and you say, both are right. How can both persons be right?

Answer: BOTH persons are right. He, who thinks negatively, sends a negative signal down to his subconsious, and his best friend and helper does his bidding, and it does not work. He, who thinks positively, sends a positive signal down to his subconscious, and his best friend and helper does his bidding, and it works. BOTH persons are right. So you see it is far better to think positively because then you create the desired positive results.

Question: They pretend, the Coué-method works instantaneously, as soon as you utter a saying, it will be fulfilled. Is that true?

Answer: No, it doesn't work this way, usually. For this method is new to the beginner. That means, it is new as well to his subconscious to get new positive orders. Your best friend and helper is used to poor old thinking. It must get accustomed to new orders and to new thinking.

Question: How much time will it require the personal subconscious to accept and realize new positive orders?

Answer: That's a question of training. He who is used to this method will find success within two or three nights. But, although being used to it, you need at least one night till your subconscious realizes your wishes.

Question: And how much time will it take the beginner?

Answer: You must consider up to three weeks to realize the first positive results. But never lay off the Coué sayings, for success is absolute sure in 70 % of all cases!

Question: I have a lot of friends. We talk all things over. What can I tell them about this method?

Answer: You must consider their possible reaction. They are not informed, because for instance there is nothing on television. They maybe would show a negative reaction.

Question: I won't mind that. Where is the problem?

Answer: The problem is with you. When you doubt it, your subconscious doubts, too. And stops working in this respect.

Question: So, what is the condition of my subconscious working effectively for me?

Answer: You must know or believe it is working. Then it works perfectly within the margin of its possiblities. Doubt stops it. Doubt destroys your knowledge or conviction."

Question: They say, the Coué-method can work miracles. For instance, I lose a leg due to an accident. Can I grow my leg again, using a positive saying?

Answer: Coué explains that any idea which we can succeed in having the subconscious accept will be realized in action, provided, however, that it is within the realms of the possible; for he realizes that the human body has limitations. Coué does not attempt the impossible. When promising benefits, he always says, 'providing this thing be possible'. So some animals could grow their lost leg, but not mankind.

Question: This is a method of wish saying?

Answer: Yes, it is. But there is an enormous power within us to fulfill each wish if ever possible.

Question: If I wish a handful of gold nuggets shall fall down from the sky in front of my feet. Does this happen?

Answer: No, this cannot happen, not this way. Due to Emile Coué, please consider only things in the sphere of possibility.

Question: So this method of wishing and wanting and of belief is nonsense?

Answer: No, on the contrary. Defeating cancer this way - wishing and wanting and demanding - is more worth than all gold of the world.

Question: If somebody is altogether healthy and sound today. Can this person do without the Coué method?

Answer: No. The Coué method prevents all diseases within the range of 70 %. So if this person wants to stay healthy and sound, he should use this method as a means of prevention. Using this wonderful method, you never get knowledge of all diseases your are avoiding this way.

Question: Hearing of the ideas Monsieur Coué is proposing, I think they are too good to be true?

Answer: The Coué method is simple. But all great things are simple. This method is simplest, so it is greatest.

Question: Does the Coué method work in each language, no matter what is the country of your origin?

Answer: The subconscious, of course, understands each person, no matter which language. Here Coué's main saying in five languages:

English: "Day by day, in all respects, I get better and better."
German: "Es geht mir mit jedem Tag in jeder Hinsicht immer besser und besser."
French: "Tous les jours, à tous points de vue, je vais de mieux en mieux."
Italian: "Ogni giorno, sotto tutti i rapporti, io vado di bene in meglio."
Spanish: "Todos los dias desde todos los puntos de vista, ya voy de mejor a mejor."

6. Ella Boyce Kirk

Ella Boyce Kirk: "My Pilgrimage to Coué" (1922).

Out of this book the following quotations:

"There always existed that enthusiasm that comes with success - and Coué's method, as I discovered later, in affections that did not entail organic malformations or broken bones, was successful in ninety cases out of one hundred." (p. 3 f)

"In all cases where the Coué method was tried, the attitude was one of satisfaction and gratitude. The individual radiated a desire to spread the idea and inform the world of the wonders that could be accomplished by a method so simple that it might at first seem ridiculous." (p. 4)

"The truth of Coué's marvelous method has in it the very essence of sunlight in its goodness and beneficence. If only it were as widely diffused how much happier the world would be!" (p. 5)

"I had reached the stage when I was about to resign myself to the worst, when the names Coué and Nancy came to me like two good geniuses leading me to health and happiness. I was not long in availing myself of the promises they held out to me, and now, thanks to them, I am able to publish my thankfulness and gratitude to the world instead of dragging my life away in embittered invalidism in the narrow confines of a basket-chair." (p. 5 f)

"... the doctor ... He told me that I was shortly going to be unable to walk!" (p. 14)

"approximately fifteen years I had suffered occasionally with both limbs from a malady that seemed to be due to gradual stiffening of the muscles. It was sometimes attended by cramps the knees. Any difficulty in walking that I experienced in this way, however, was always attributed not only by my doctor, but even by myself, to the fact that I was so heavy." (p. 15)

"One day, most unexpectedly, the trouble I had experienced with my knees showed new developments that seemed grave enough to demand serious attention. Pains so intense as to cause me to lose all consciousness, and swellings so gross as to interfere with my walking challenged notice. The doctors came and diagnosed. One said dropsy; another, rheumatism. All decreed that probably, at my time of life, it was incurable. With rest and diet I would perhaps bring about reduction of the swelling, but it was nevertheless probably futile to expect that I should again walk with the old freedom." (p. 16)

"But illness is most often mental. Indeed, it ought to be borne in mind by those who are well that no invalidism is unbearable if it is cheered by

23

employment, interesting company, and a chance to render service. The chief duty of those who nurse the sick is to restore their mental health." (p. 22 f)

"Looking back upon my decision to go to M. Coué, it seems to me as if it came as a last resort, when despair had all but set it." (p. 23)

"Accordingly, we set sail on the 8th of July. Established in a special deck chair that had been built expressly to accomodate my poor, tortured body, I vowed not to leave it unless I was washed out to sea by a tidal wave." (p. 24)

"... I had already tried several varieties of religious faith cures. At this moment I have nothing to urge against them. In the light of my subsequent lessons from M. Coué, I have more respect for them now than before I went to him, for he convinced me that they are of value for many people. His explanation that they are sometimes efficacious because they often cause the patient to give himself curative autosuggestions justifies them for those who can be convinced by their affirmations. However, they failed to help me, because I had no faith in them." (p. 25)

"We had not been long in his study when M. Coué entered. How shall I depict him in words? Sixty-seven years young, short in stature, with a remarkably keen eye and a twinkling smile, he appears at first glance to be bent with age, but one flash of his merry smile instantly sets that impression to rest. One feels, to begin with, how unassuming he is; next, how sincere; and lastly, how assured. 'You will be better', seems to be his most characteristic remark." (p. 33)

"Coué: 'If, then, the patient acts on these he will get well, if it is within the limits of possibility.'" (p. 35)

"He explained later that if the disease of the eye is a muscular one, he can cure it, but if there are liquid complications, he cannot." (p. 35)

"My personal experience in being treated by Monsieur Coué is so simple as to be unbelievable..." (p. 37)

"Even then I did not believe it possible; it all seemed so simple as to be only a passing fancy. I repeated twenty times every morning and evening, as he asked me to do, 'Day by day, in every way, I am getting better und better', sometimes adding, 'and I am sure there will be no recurrence of the pain.' M. Coué said there was no objection to making this specific suggestion, though it was not at all necessary. In less than a week I found that I could move about more easily and could do more things without conscious effort than I had been able to do for years. It was then that the real cure was effected. I could now sit for a long time without changing position. I could walk much more easily and after three months, during which time I have surely been getting better and better each day, there has been no recurrence of the pain and I walk as well and as easily as I did twenty years ago. - The method that brought about this result seems almost too simple to tell." (p. 38 f)

24

"Precisely what you suffered from was not so much a disease as a moral disaster; the cure has given you more than the absence of pain. Something positive has been gained - what M. Coué calls 'Self-Mastery'. You are led to see that life has more spiritual value than you had given heed to." (p. 40)

"It needs but a glance to see what has brought them hither; faces drawn with pain, the tortured look of mental distress, the twisted and bent frames supported by cane or crutch, all bear silent testimony to the need and the hope of relief." (p. 42)

"... it minimizes the possiblities of the patient's discussion of his own symptoms. To dwell upon symptoms is to make a suggestion, which is highly undesirable. We all know how characteristic it is to rehearse symptoms, particularly in the case of chronic invalids. However, in a large group it becomes practically impossible, and that is a first step toward eliminating an evil suggestion and substituting a good one." (p. 43)

"M. Coué, as is well known, maintains that the imagination [subconscious] is stronger than the will." (p. 45)

"First of all, let us consider what the unconscious does for us. There are many bodily und mental activities which we can consciously direct and alter; but there are many more, of greater importance, that we cannot control through the mind. These are more important because they are the fundamental life activities without which life could not continue. Breathing, the beating of the heart, the processes of digestion and many more, all come under that category." (p. 48)

"It has remained for M. Coué to discover the real nature of the unconscious, and to present it not as an evil genius, rising from the depths from time to time under emotional impulsion to defeat our most earnest purposes; but that it is a deep and vital force, capable of being educated and directed, provided that the laws under which it works are observed." (p. 50)

"... the subconscious ... It is well known that it is during sleep that it is most active." (p. 51)

"M. Coué, therefore, advocates that upon retiring, and also immediately upon waking, while the mind and body are as relaxed as possible, everyone should make to himself the general suggestion of well-being that is coming to be a household expression: 'Day by day, in every way, I am getting better and better.' This is to be said twenty times. M. Coué also suggests the use of a string with twenty knots tied to it, for keeping the record, and the uttering of the words in as monotonous a tone as possible. In other words, what is known in psychology as voluntary or active attention should be reduced to a minimum; the conscious self is to be lulled to as quiescent a state as possible, short of actual sleep. M. Coué explains that any idea which we can succeed in having the subconscious accept will be realized in action, provided, however, that it is within the realms of the possible; for he realizes that the human body has limitations." (p. 51 f)

"A second important thing is his method of repetition. ... It is used extensively in the business world, and advertising has built a scientific law about it." (p. 53)

"In his various clinics M. Coué has conquered cases of paralysis, tuberculosis, asthma, anaemia, stuttering, enteritis, gout, dyspepsia, eczema and neurasthenia in all its manifestations. The crippled have thrown away their crutches und walked for the first time, sometimes after a single treatment." (p. 62)

"Christian Scientists, when they achieve similar results, assert that it is divine healing. Those in charge of Catholic shrines such as Lourdes and Ste. Anne de Beaupré say that it is God working through the intercession of particular saints in special localities that produces the marvelous results. Hindoo healers have claimed magical or religious powers to cure, in similar fashion. Even the proof of Christ's own divinity is sometimes asserted on the strength of the miracles of healing which He performed. - The popular mind is thoroughly prepared to believe that divine power can produce particular cures, that the Deity does sometimes take note of, and miraculously heal individuals, and that the possession, therefore, by a human being, of power to effect cures in an unexplained fashion without material aid is in itself proof of his possessing some superhuman, spiritual force." (p. 62 f)

"Not his personal power, but autosuggestion conveyed by the subject himself, to himself, is Coué's own explanation for his cures. Autosuggestion he defines as a sort of self-hypnotism, 'the influence of the imagination upon the moral und physical being'. - 'If you persuade yourself that you can do a certain thing, provided that thing be possible, you will do it, however difficult it may be.' - To one patient Coué said: 'When I tell you that you are better, you do feel better at once, don't you? Why? Because you have faith in me. Just believe in yourself and you will obtain the same result.'" (p. 66 f)

"'When certain people do not obtain satisfactory results with autosuggestion, it is either because they lack confidence, or because they make efforts, which is the more frequent case. To make good suggestions it is absolutely necessary to do so without effort. Conscious autosuggestion, made with confidence, with faith, with perseverance, realizes itself mathematically, without reason.' - Coué, then, lays no claim to personal power, or even religious aid in effecting cures. Indeed, as we have seen, he ascribes to autosuggestion the cures for which religious sanction is asserted. - 'The means employed by the healers all go back to autosuggestion', he says. 'That is to say, that these methods, whatever they are - words, incantations, gestures, staging - all produce in the patient the autosuggestion of recovery.'" (p. 67 f)

"What genius it reveals, after all, to take a few simple instruments, such as a string of twenty knots, a doggerel of twelve words, and two or three easy affirmations, and to create out of them a system of drugless medicine that has the world at respectful attention!" (p. 73)

"The hardest thing for most people to understand about Couéism is that there isn't more of it. The sole tenet in the system is the deliberately adopted belief that, whatever ails you, your are getting better. The sole means of forming that belief is to put the affirmation to work in your subconscious mind, with the expectation that the subconscious mind will carry the belief out into actuality while you are occupied with other things. The sole means of putting that belief to work is to din it into the mind by tireless assertion at those times of day when the will is most quiescent, and when the fancy is most credulous." (p. 74)

"... a sing-song of childlike simplicity..." (p. 76)

"There are, indeed, hurdles to be got over before the subconscious mind can accept the suggestion of daily growing better. In the minds of the skeptical, doubts must be removed, suggestibility built up, hope enkindled, faith engendered, and a desire aroused sufficient to keep the subject repeating the formula long enough for it to start its work in the subconscious." (p. 77)

"He does not attempt the impossible. When promising benefits, he always says, 'providing this thing be possible'." (p. 80 f)

"'What you say persistently and very quickly comes to pass (within the domain of the reasonable, of course).'" (p. 81)

"The small percentage of insane, of people of arrested mental development are also ruled out as outside the range of his ministrations." (p. 82)

"'You say that you have suffered for forty years? It is none the less true that you can be cured to-morrow, on condition, naturally, of your doing exactly what I tell you to do, in the way I tell you to do it.'" (p. 83)

"All successful physicians nowadays recognize this fact, - that an optimistic attitude toward a disease is the first essential for a cure." (p. 84)

"The conscious attitude of confidence, hope and striving is necessary to maintain health." (p. 88)

"It is Coué's discovery that whatever idea is presented to the unconscious with an attitude of belief is accepted as reality and gradually realizes itself in the unconscious. Hence his constant mission of favorable suggestions to the unconscious." (p. 90)

7. Art and More

There is a subconscious, the greatest, godlike power in us. There are so many examples we could add to all what, above, already has been said. For instance, dear reader, you are looking for a book. It should be alphabetically listed on the shelf, but it is not there where it should be. Well, you think, where is it now? You do not know, but what happens then? Maybe two hours later or the next day, all of a sudden, you know where this book is and why you changed its place.

You see, your subconscious always is working, day and night. Your best friend and helper provides you with the necessary information of which you are thinking: "Oh, yes, it was my idea!" But no, it was not your idea, it was your subconscious (never forgetting anything) providing you with the place where the missed book must be.

Another example. We so often are searching for a name or a word we would like to mention this moment - in a discussion or just thinking of it. But the word or name are insistently missing. Please mind you, missing it is only for your "I". Your subconscious has no problems with it because your subconscious memorizes everything and never will forget all of these memories. So try it without any exertion or just wait some time and soon your best friend and helper will provide you with the word or name you so urgently are missing.

Now, please mind, as we have already told, your personal subconscious is partially independent and it is acting on its own! That means it does things you never dreamt of, and it is assisting you in all your yearning. Say, you are an author writing a book or a story, then your mind is busy with contents, but your subconscious is busy as well. You got a problem here, you got a problem there? The solution, you will find it! But, again, it is a very wrong estimation neglecting the role your subconscious played in finding that solution. So, maybe considering the author of MacBeth and Hamlet, we should read: written by William Shakespeare AND his subconscious!

In art and literature there are many examples of authors or composers saying their ideas were coming over night (when the personal subconscious has all time to work on it). Let us take a well known example out of the area of the fantastic. Let us l isten to what Robert Louis Stevenson, creator of the famous novel "The Strange Case of Dr. Jekyll and Mr. Hyde", said insofar:

"But to use your mind to the best advantage doesn't mean to toil along with the mere conscious part of it. It means hitching up your conscious mind with the Man Inside You, with the little 'Mental Brownies' as Robert Louis Stevenson called them, and then working together for a definite end.

'My Brownies! God bless them!' said Stevenson, 'Who do one-half of my work for me when I am fast asleep, and in all human likelihood do the rest for me as well when I am wide awake and foolishly suppose that I do it myself. I had long been wanting to write a book on man's double being. For two days I went about racking my brain for a plot of any sort, and on the second night I dreamt the scene in Dr. Jekyll and Mr. Hyde at the window; and a scene, afterward split in two, in which Hyde, pursued, took the powder and underwent the change in the presence of his pursuer.' ...

'In the Inner Consciousness of each of us', quotes Dumont in 'The Master

Mind', 'there are forces which act much the same as would countless tiny mental brownies or helpers who are anxious and willing to assist us in our mental work, if we will but have confidence and trust in them. This is a psychological truth expressed in the terms of old fairy tales.'"
(Robert Collier: The Secret of the Ages, p. 50)

These "brownies" exist as well in German fairy tales. Here they are called "Heinzelmännchen" (his good helpers). There someone goes to bed, without having done his work. But the "Heinzelmännchen" do all his work during the night, and when he awakes, fine, the shop is done. The fairy tale refers to work done by hand. But in reality, as you can see above, the helpers do their work in your head and in your soul!
Does the subconscious only work for artists, writers, composers and so on? No, of course not. It, the personal subconscious, is an attribute of all women and men, and everywhere in nature it is present. It works best at night, as we have seen above, because at daytime it is busy with so much ado, but at night time the eager "I" comes to a rest, so it is time for the subconscious to solve the bottled up problems.
Look at this quotation here:
"Frederick Pierce, in 'Our Unconscious Mind', gives an excellent method for solving business problems through the aid of the subconscious:
'Several years ago, I heard a successful executive tell a group of young men how he did his work, and included in the talk was the advice to prepare at the close of each day's business, a list of the ten most important things for the next day. To this I would add: Run them over in the mind just before going to sleep, not thoughtfully, or with elaboration of detail, but with the sure knowledge that the deeper centers of the mind are capable of viewing them constructively even though conscious attention is surrendered in sleep.
'Then, if there is a particular problem which seems difficult of solution, review its features lightly as a last game for the imaginative unconscious to play at during the night. Do not be discouraged if no immediate results are apparent. Remember that fiction, poetry, musical composition, inventions, innumerable ideas, spring from the unconscious, often in forms that give evidence of the highest constructive elaboration.
'Give your unconscious a chance. Give it the material, and stimulate it with keenly dwelt-on wishes along frank Ego Maximation lines. It is a habit which, if persisted in, will sooner or later present you with some very valuable ideas when you least expect them.'"
(Robert Collier: The Secret of the Ages, p. 120)

8. Final Quotations

There is so much to it, to the subconscious, we do never notice. Mind you, your hairs are growing on your head, your finger nails grow as well. Did you way of your "I" ever waste any thought on it? No, you never did. But they are growing anyway. Or take your hidden inner organs of which you maybe even do not know the name? Hopefully they work for you best. Each organ works in cooperation with all the others. That is like an orchestra where a lot of instruments are playing together. But you immediately realize: regarding to an orchestra, you need a conductor so that all instruments will sound together very well. But what about your body, and its organs? Who is the conductor there, so that all organs fit together? Yes, there must be a conductor whom we just do not realize, subconscious is his name.

There are a lot of things unthought of. Finally in this text let us have a look at what Shakespeare and so many others considered, referring to the secret power within us, which only a part of God can be.

"This field is your own consciousness - a treasure you find within yourself -, which others cannot see. But you know it for the in-dwelling Spirit - 'the Father within you' - and are willing to sell all that you have because this treasure is worth more than all other possessions.

"If you have begun to realize this treasure, and use it even in a small way, the most wonderful thing that can happen to anyone on this planet has happened to you."

(Robert Collier: "The Secret of the Ages", p. 161)

"Even as long ago as Napoleon's day, men had begun to get an inkling of this. 'Think that you are well,' said the astute Tallyrand, 'instead of thinking that you are sick.' And the formula of the Quakers is that an energetic soul is 'master of the body which it loves.'"

(Robert Collier: The Secret of the Ages, p. 152)

"Few sick people have any idea how much they can do for themselves. There is an old saying that every man is 'a fool or his own physician at 40.'"

(Robert Collier: The Secret of the Ages, p. 153)

"What image are you holding in mind? Images of sickness? Of poverty? Of Limitation? Then you are reproducing these in your life. Banish them! Forget them! Never let them enter your thought, and they will never again manifest themselves in your life."

(Robert Collier: The Secret of the Ages, p. 153

Oh yes, did you ever hear the voice of God within you? No? Why don't you listen carefully, ignoring the loud troubling noise outside you?

"That is a great sentiment which was expressed by Fénelon. He said: 'We must lend an attentive ear, for God's voice is soft and still, and is only heard by those who hear nothing else. Ah! how rare it is to find a soul still enough

to hear God speak.'"
(Henry Wood: "Edward Burton", p. 260)

Or listen to this, regarding the fact that words are not useless, but a powerful force:

"Sticks and stones will break my bones ... but words will drive me crazy. Be careful of the words you use!"
(Barbara Ruth Hailey quotes her teacher Alice Ginott, from: INTA-Magazine "New Thought" Issue Autumn 2015, p. 29)

And what about William Shakespeare, the greatest author and poet ever?

"As A Man Thinketh

Our remedies in ourselves do lie
Which we ascribe to heaven."
                    Shakespeare
(Robert Collier: "The Secret of the Ages", p. 59)

Well, what about your age? You are too old to consider what all these great women and men have thought? No, you are not at all too old, listen to this, Berton Braley has it well expressed in his poem on 'Opportunity':

            "For the best verse hasn't been rhymed yet,
The best house hasn't been planned,
The highest peak hasn't been climbed yet,
The mightiest rivers aren't spanned.

Don't worry and fret, faint hearted,
The chances have just begun,
For the Best jobs haven't been started,
The Best work hasn't been done."
(Robert Collier: The Secret of the Ages, p. 68)

Well, now, we understand this: we, well considered, are the masters of our fate.

            "It matters not how strait the gate,
How charged with punishment the scroll,
I am the Master of my Fate,
I am the Captain of my Soul."
Henley
(Robert Collier: "The Secret of the Ages", p. 15)

And finally, please, let us have a look at a very fine quotation which shows us the ways God goes without our often noticing it:

>All the prophets in heaven were gathered together trying to decide where

to hide the secrets of life so that man would never find them. One of the prophets spoke up, "We will hide them far out in outer-space". But God said that man would go to the furthest corner of outer-space and would find the secrets of life. Another prophet suggested that the secrets be hidden deep in the ocean. God exclaimed: "Man would also go to the depths of the deepest ocean and he would find them". The prophets then questioned, "Where will we hide the secrets of life so man can't find them"? God's loving voice replied, "We will hide them within Man himself - he will never look".<
(From INTA-Magazine "New Thought" Issue Autumn 2015, p. 28, quoted by Rev. Barbara Ruth Hailey)